GOUT

MW01242541

Containing Gout Cookbook
Cooking With Spices for Gout Relief
&
50 Gout Relief Smoothie Recipes
With 10 Day Meal Plan Guide
& More

HR Research Alliance

Legal & Disclaimer

The information contained in this book and its contents is not designed to replace or take the place of any form of medical or professional advice; and is not meant to replace the need for independent medical, financial, legal or other professional advice or services, as may be required. The content and information in this book has been provided for educational and entertainment purposes only.

The content and information contained in this book has been compiled from sources deemed reliable, and it is accurate to the best of the Author's knowledge, information and belief. However, the Author cannot guarantee its accuracy and validity and cannot be held liable for any errors and/or omissions. Further, changes are periodically made to this book as and when needed. Where appropriate and/or necessary, you must consult a professional (including but not limited to your doctor, attorney, financial advisor or such other professional advisor) before using any of the suggested remedies, techniques, or information in this book.

Upon using the contents and information contained in this book, you agree to hold harmless the Author from and against any damages, costs, and expenses, including any legal fees potentially resulting from the application of any of the information provided by this book. This disclaimer applies to any loss, damages or injury caused by the use and application, whether directly or indirectly, of any advice or information presented, whether for breach of contract, tort, negligence, personal injury, criminal intent, or under any other cause of action.

You agree to accept all risks of using the information presented inside this book.

You agree that by continuing to read this book, where appropriate and/or necessary, you shall consult a professional (including but not limited to your doctor, attorney, or financial advisor or such other advisor as needed) before using any of the suggested remedies, techniques, or information in this book.

Contents

Refreshing Classic: Oranges, Apple, Grape 104

Banana Bahama Mama: Banana, Pineapple, Orange 105

Orange Power: Orange, Carrot, Turmeric 106

What a Plummy Pear: Plum, Pear, Blueberry 107

Merry Berries and Plum: Cherry, Strawberry, Plum 108

Apple Pie: Apple, Cinnamon, Almond 109

Beet the Rush Smoothie: Beet, Strawberry, Raspberry 110

Watermelon-Basil Lemonade: Watermelon, Strawberry, Basil 111

Creamy Cantaloupe: Cantaloupe, Pineapple, Banana 112

Peary-Cherry: Pear, Cherry 113

Peaches and Green: Peach & Avocado 114

Sweet Potato Pie: Sweet potato & Banana 115

Sweet Peach Tea: Peach, Green Tea 116

Sparkling Peach Spritzer: Peach, Grape 117

Cherry Citrus Smoothie: Pineapple, Cherry 118

Sunrise Smoothie: Kiwi, Watermelon, Strawberry 119

Better Birthday Cake: Vanilla, Spinach, Banana 120

Blue Raspberry Tea: Blueberry, Raspberry, White Tea 121

Blackberry Mango Tango: Blackberry, Mango, Honeydew 122

Mango Berry Smoothie: Mango, Blueberry 123

You've Broc-To Be Kidding: Broccoli, Blueberry, Orange 124

Blackberry Cobbler: Blackberry, Almond 125

Lean, Mean, and Green: Spinach, Celery, Kiwi 126

P. B. & Green: Banana, Peanut butter, Spinach 127

Very Berry Cranberry: Raspberry, Cranberry 128

Feel the Beet: Banana & Beet 129

Super Booster Smoothie: Cranberry, Blueberry, Kale 130

Cauli-berry Smoothie: Strawberry, Cherry, Cauliflower 131

Pumpkin Pie Smoothie: Pumpkin, Banana, Cinnamon 132

Better Bloody Mary: Tomato, Strawberry, Basil 133

Papaya Creamsicle Smoothie: Papaya, Carrot, Banana 134

Avo-Cacao Smoothie: Avocado, Peanut Butter, Cacao 135

Green and Blue: Avocado, Blueberry, Spinach 136

A.K.C. Champion Smoothie: Avocado, Kiwi, Cucumber 137

Watermelon Sparkler: Watermelon, Cucumber, Lemon 138

Lemon Drop Smoothie: Lemon & Cucumber 139

Sweet Shirley Temple: Cherry, Orange, Ginger 140

P.B & K: Pineapple, Blueberry, Kale 141

Purple Power Punch: Red Cabbage, Cherry, Blackberry 142

Pina Caul-ada-flour Smoothie: Cauliflower, Pineapple, Orange 143

Hibiscus Citrus Quencher: Hibiscus Tea, Orange, Strawberry 144

Spiced Orange Smoothie: Orange, Turmeric, Cinnamon 145

Pineapple Zinger: Pineapple, Ginger 146

Maximum Mango Smoothie: Mango, Cayenne, Strawberry 147

Lettuce Be Cherry: Romaine Lettuce, Blueberry, Cherry 148

The Ultimate Cress: Watercress, Apple, Avocado 149

Dressed to Dill: Cucumber, Spinach, Dill 150

Black Forest Cake: Cherry, Banana, Almond 151

Spiced Carrot Cake: Carrot, Almond, Cinnamon 152

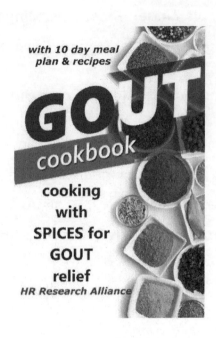

Waking up to gout is frightening and painful. You went to bed fine the night before and you wake up one morning to an unimaginable pain. You may be suffering from just a swollen big toe, or you may have all over joint pain. However gout affects you, all you want is relief from the pain. While your doctor may have prescribed anti-inflammatories, there can be remedies right in the very foods that you eat to help you through this difficult time. Since they are food related, you may not even have to worry about food/drug interactions and may be able to use them side-by-side in your treatment plan. Just remember to talk to your doctor about any herbal or food related choices just to be safe!

Let's take a quick look at gout itself and then we will share some spices and other foods that help to bring relief and healing from a gout attack.

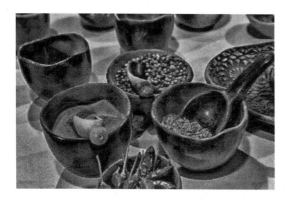

Gouty Arthritis Explained

Gout is a quick onset type of arthritis that hits you suddenly. Or so you may think. You see, when your first attack of gout hits the uric acid levels that cause the attack have been rising in your body for quite some time. Uric acid is a "by-product" of purine in the foods that you eat. Foods that contain purines include; cured meat, organ meat, dried legumes, beer, canned fish, and heavy gravies made from meat juices and fats. If you have risk factors for gout, your body is unable to break down and properly excrete purines via the kidneys and turns them into high levels of uric acid. High levels of uric acid in your blood is called, hyperuricemia.

Gout pain comes from excessive levels of uric acid turning into crystals that settle in the soft tissues near the joints in your body. Most often, the first attack occurs in the joints surrounding your large or great toe. Crystals rubbing on the joints and soft tissue leads to inflammation, swelling, and pain. Gout is often felt in the great toe, elbow joints, fingers, ankles, wrists, and knees.

If gout continues untreated, the uric acid crystals may even build up and you may notice small bumps just under the skin around your joints and even in your earlobes. These bumps are known as, tophi. Uric acid crystals may also get stuck in your kidneys and form kidney stones. Tophi have also been found in the lungs and eyes. Because of these complications, early evaluation and treatment is very important.

Gout tends to occur in "flares" and may last from days to even weeks. The flares tend to subside and go away, but may occur over and over again. Unlike rheumatoid arthritis where the symptoms are present on a daily basis, gout symptoms are only present during a flare. This may lead to a false sense of security that gout is gone and people may stop prevention and treatment measures thinking gout is no longer present. However, once you have had one gout flare you are susceptible to more in the future.

The Four Gout Stages

Gout has a pattern and four distinct stages, although you may never know that you are in the first stage of gout. It is almost completely silent. The other stages are more pronounced. Once again it is important to know if you are at risk for gout, so you can begin preventative measures early on. Here are the stages:

Stage One: Silent or Asymptomatic Gout

This stage is silently occurring right under your nose. There could never be a more perfect time to add healing spices to your diet. Look for things that help control uric acid levels and improve kidney function. This stage usually does not have any symptoms, but the uric acid levels are rising from the things that you eat.

Stage Two: Acute Gout Attack

Stage two is actually the onset of a gout attack, with severe pain. Crystals from high uric acid levels are now damaging the soft tissues near and in your joints. While you should see your doctor for evaluation and treatment, there are spices that may bring you relief during this intense stage of pain and inflammation. Spices may also help prevent a second or subsequent attack and shorten the course. Make sure to mention this to your doc.

Stage 3: Remission Period

After the first acute flare subsides, you may be feeling great again! While the symptoms have gone away, you still are considered a gout sufferer. At this time, you will really want to "step up your game." You may not be in pain, but your body is still having a hard time controlling uric acid levels. This is another important time for preventative measures, like using spices that can control inflammation and uric acid in your cooking.

Final Stage: Chronic Gout

Hopefully, you can reverse this stage with good care and preventative measures. Gout that is not fully treated can turn into chronic gout with recurrent attacks. If left untreated or undertreated, gout may cause permanent joint damage.

Gout Statistics

Gout is believed to affect more than 8 million people in the United States. Another 21 percent of the population has been found to have higher uric acid levels in their blood, putting them at risk for gout. If only they knew ways to manage this stage of the disease before it gets out of hand.

If you have risk factors for gout, it is a good idea to have your uric acid levels checked at your yearly physical. This way you can begin "gout prevention" measures to help ward off an attack. This could include eating foods made with spices that help keep uric acid and inflammation levels under control. This brings up the question, "what are the risk factors for gout?"

Risk Factors for Gout

The journey begins with knowing if you have risk factors for gout. Gout has multiple risk factors, the same as other types of arthritis. While a large portion of acquiring gout is due to poor diet, there is also a large underlying portion that is attributed to other things. These factors include:

- Alcohol Use (Beer)
- Diet High in Purines (Organ Meats, Gravies, Seafood, High Fructose)
- Family History of Gout
- Hypertension
- Diuretic Use
- Diabetes
- Obesity
- High Cholesterol
- Male Gender (Females are also at risk)
- Middle Age

One of the strongest of these factors is, obesity. Coupled with diabetes and hypertension can be a gold ticket to a gout flare. Obesity can increase the amount of pain you feel with attacks due to pressure on the affected joints. Obesity with the addition of high blood sugar can put a strain on the kidneys, reducing their ability to lower uric acid levels in the blood.

Symptoms of Gout

In order to get evaluated and begin early prevention in treatment, you should know the symptoms of a gout attack. This will help you recognize what is going on early in the game so you can take the steps to bring things under control. Symptoms of gout include:

- Joint Pain (Especially in the big toe)

- Pain and Discomfort in more than one joint

- Swelling, Inflammation and Heat

- Low-Grade Fevers

- Redness to the Skin

- Stiff Joints

- Itchy Skin

- Tophi aka Nodules under the skin near the affected joints

- Immobility

Any of these symptoms should be evaluated by a doctor as soon as possible. If you wake up in the morning with one swollen and red great toe with severe pain, seek medical attention that same day. This is a classic gout symptom with the onset of acute attacks.

Gout Diagnosis and Treatment

If you are at risk for gout, you can ask your doctor to check your uric acid levels at your yearly physical. This is important before you feel the pain of the first attack. You can start preventative measures right away and hopefully ward off an attack. Some preventative measures may include:

- Dietary Changes Eliminating High Purine Foods

- Reduction of Alcohol Use

- Increased Water Intake

- Increase Certain Spices in your Diet

- Exercise and Weight Loss

- Controlling Diabetes and Hypertension

If you are already suffering an initial acute attack of gout, your doctor will run necessary blood tests and possibly x-rays or an MRI to check the soft tissue near the joints. He or she may prescribe treatments to bring the attack under control. These may include:

- Anti-Inflammatory Medications

- Uric Acid Reducing Medications

- Diet Low in Purines

- Weight Loss

- Increased Exercise

- Extra Water Intake

- Rest Until Inflammation Subsides

20 Spices That May Relieve Gout

The good news is, when you have gout you have the option of many anti-inflammatory spices that can be included in your cooking to help relieve symptoms and lower uric acid levels. While you may be planning the foods you eat during mealtimes, what is equally important is the spices you use to cook your meals.

Dietary researchers have found that foods can cause inflammation in the body, or decrease inflammation in the body depending on the food. Some foods trigger your body to release chemicals that reduce inflammation, and some increase your body's production of prostaglandins, the chemicals that cause inflammation.

It is believed that if you add anti-inflammatory spices to your cooking, you can help prevent your body from releasing prostaglandins. People often don't realize that certain spices are very helpful in lowering inflammation levels in the body. In any arthritis type condition, spices should be added to cooking throughout the day for steady and ongoing relief. Even starting with some cinnamon on oatmeal in the morning, curried soups for lunch, and ending the day with fresh basil tossed into a bowl of pasta at dinner. The spices may be minimal each meal, but the benefits add up over the course of the day.

Now that we know the best ways to use them in cooking, let's take a look at some of the top anti-inflammatory and pain relieving spices for gout relief:

1. Cinnamon

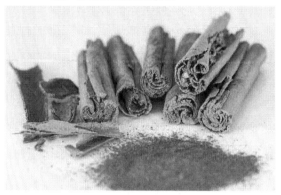

Cinnamon is a delicious and popular spice that can be used in both sweet and savory dishes for a spicy flavor. It contains cinnamic aldehyde and cinnamyl aldehydeis, which studies show these chemicals have anti-inflammatory properties. The effects are mild, but pack a good punch against inflammation when combined with another spice or food that has the same properties.

Try sprinkling some cinnamon on your hot or cold cereal in the morning. Use a dash in hot soups for lunch or dinner and use in hot beverages for extra flavor. The more often you use it during the day, the benefits will add up over time.

2. Garlic

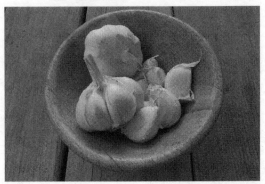

Garlic gives your food an amazing flavor and aroma, plus is versatile and can be used in any of your savory dishes. The anti-inflammatory chemical is diallyl disulfide, that reduces cytokines. Cytokines are one of the substances that increase inflammation in the body. Garlic is also a powerful antioxidant and has pain relieving properties.
The best way to eat garlic for its gout relieving properties is to use is freshly crushed into your foods. It is best crushed from raw cloves, as processed or dried garlic have weaker properties. Try some in your favorite pasta sauces, crushed

over chicken before roasting, or stirred into hummus dip.

3. Cayenne Pepper

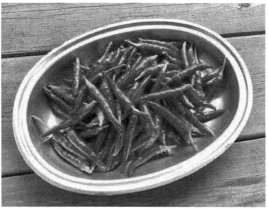

Cayenne peppers have a chemical known as, capsaicin. This has pain relieving properties by causing the body to release a chemical called, substance P. When the capsaicin enters the body or touches the skin it causes a slight burning sensation. Your body perceives this as pain and releases the substance P to signal the body to release its own pain relieving chemicals.

Cayenne is best in hispanic type foods, chili beans, and even rubbed on meats before cooking. You can also add a dash to potato salads or even soups. Always use it sparingly as it can be very spicy. Using it over the course of the day will help build-up pain relieving properties. You can also make a rub to use directly on your skin over the affected joints.

4. Turmeric

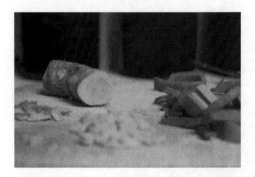

Turmeric is actually a root that contains a chemical known as, curcumin. This is a powerful anti-inflammatory that can actually block cytokines that cause inflammation. It also blocks other enzymes that cause inflammation in the body. It has been proven effective in several studies, with reduced swelling and pain in the joints.

Turmeric works best in Indian style foods and curries. Using it in combination with black pepper helps absorption. It will give foods a bright yellow color and adds a nice spicy touch to many different foods.

5. Ginger

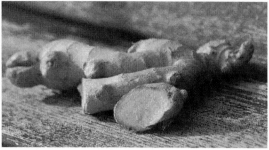

Ginger is a very popular remedy for many things including, inflammation. It contains both shogaol and gingerol that block the body's response to chemicals that cause inflammation. It may also have pain relieving benefits.

Ginger can be used in your savory foods as well as sweet foods. Use this root freshly chopped or ground for best results. You can even make it into a cup of tea with some honey and lemon. Ginger root may be effective for joint pain by making a paste and applying it directly to the skin over the affected joint.

6. Celery Seed

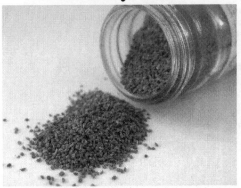

Celery seeds contain 3-n-Butylpthalidewhich, a potent diuretic that can increase the body's ability to flush out toxins like, uric acid. It makes your kidneys pull the uric acid from your blood and excrete it into your urine. It also helps to make your blood more alkaline. They have also been found to be rich in Omega 6 fatty acids and other powerful anti-inflammatory agents to help reduce inflammation and pain in the body.

Celery seeds can be sprinkled on salads or used in curry type dishes. It can be a very strong and bitter tasting spice, but used sparingly can add a nice touch to your spicy, savory dishes. You can also make it into a tea that you drink throughout the day.

7. Parsley

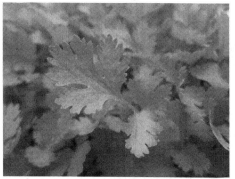

Parsley contains quercetin and kaempferol, which may help reduce levels of uric acid in the body. Parsley has natural diuretic properties to help your kidneys flush out toxins and may even help prevent kidney stones. It also contains a flavonoid known as, apigenin that reduces the body's ability to convert purines to uric acid.

Parsley has a wonderful bright natural flavor that can enhance any dish during cooking. It also makes a nice garnish that refreshes the breath and calms the stomach when chewed raw after meals.

8. Thyme

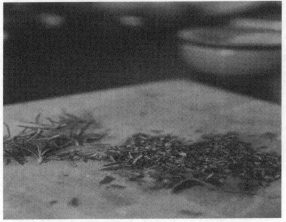

Thyme is another spice that contains high levels of, apigenin. This chemical can really help reduce the production of uric acid in the body from purines in the diet. Thyme also contains, carvacrol, which is a natural anti-inflammatory.

Thyme is good with chicken dishes, in soups, and stuffings used in poultry. You can also use thyme to make an effective tea for gout relief.

9. Basil

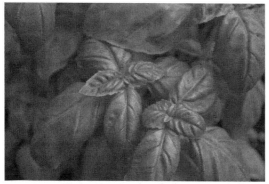

Basil contains a volatile oil called, eugenol. This chemical blocks cyclooxygenase or COX that increases inflammation during gout attacks. Eugenol works similar to NSAID's and pain relievers by blocking the action of COX.

Basil works great rubbed on meats, used in sauces, and even sprinkled in a salad.

10.   Clove

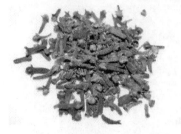

Cloves contain both apigenin and eugenol making them both helpful to lower uric acid levels and relieve inflammation. They are tasty in both sweet and savory foods when used in small amounts. They add a tasty twist to hams, spice cakes, spiked into an onion in stews, and steeped into a hot tea.

11.   Coriander Seed/Cilantro

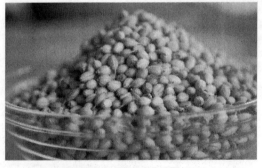

Coriander seed is actually the seed for the leafy green plant, cilantro. It contains two flavanoids, apigenin and rutin that were shown in small studies to help lower uric acid levels. It wasn't shown to have much of an anti-inflammatory effect, but can be paired with other spices that reduce inflammation.

Cilantro is a delicious addition to hispanic foods, salads, and side dishes. Coriander seed can be used as a thickener or spice in sauces and stews.

12.   Lavender

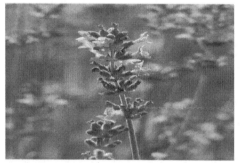

Lavender is showing signs of being a powerful anti-inflammatory. In studies that have been performed, lavender has almost the same effects as corticosteroids and prescription pain relievers. Researchers continue to look into why lavender has these effects, but the data seems very promising.

Lavender is delicious in sweet foods and desserts. It can also add an aromatic flavor to grilled shrimp, herb butter, and infused into sugar for cookies.

13.   Lemon Balm

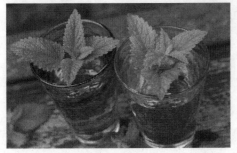

Lemon balm can have a powerful anti-inflammatory effect on the body. Two chemicals, rosmaric acid and quercetin both help lower inflammation in the body during gout attacks. Rosamric acid is also a very powerful antioxidant that may also help flush toxins out of the body like, uric acid.

Lemon balm is from the mint family and works deliciously in dessert foods, tossed into salads, and mixed into salad dressings.

14.   Liquorice Root

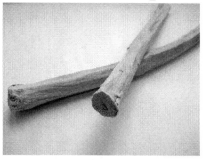

Liquorice has anti-inflammatory properties and may help relieve gout pain. It also helps block xanthine oxidase, the chemical in the body that turns purines into uric acid. Use caution with licorice because it can raise blood pressure. It is safe in small amounts.

15.   Peppermint

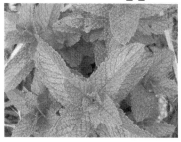

Peppermint is high in menthol oil that can help relieve gout pain. Drinking it in
tea may help reduce uric acid levels and you can rub a little on your inflamed joints for relief of inflammation and pain. Peppermint is a great seasoning for both sweet and savory dishes.

16.   Rosemary

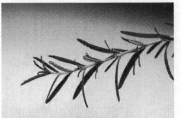

Rosemary is a strong and aromatic herb that can liven up the taste of any dish. Long used for gout, it increases circulation and helps the body get rid of uric acid. It can also reduce inflammation, redness, and the pain of gout.

Use some broken off twigs on freshly baked breads, sprinkle some in stews, or use as a garnish on hot foods. Heating rosemary will help to release the helpful oils into your foods.

17.   Nettle

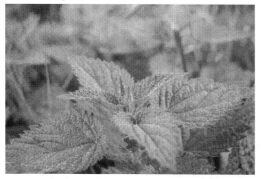

Stinging nettles may send a shiver through your spine when you think you might have to touch them. When harvested (with gloves, of course) they can be an amazing addition to things you cook. Nettle is a natural diuretic, increasing the kidneys ability to flush out uric acid from your blood.

Use garden gloves to harvest the leaves and rinse well. When you toss them into a pot of boiling water, the hairs are instantly neutralized. You may still see the hairs on the leaves, but the ability to sting is lost. Make sure you cook them well until the leaves are crisp. They work well to replace cooked spinach or even as a filler for vegetable lasagna. You can also toss it into stew, soups, or eat them sauteed.

19. Marjoram

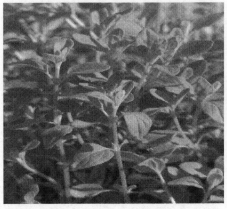

Marjoram has many different health benefits and can work as a pain reliever for joint and muscle pain. It can also help to relieve inflammation from gout. This spice also helps increase blood flow and helps to warm and soothe painful areas. The increased circulation encourages the body to clear out toxins and excess fluids. This effect may help reduce uric acid levels in the blood. It is encouraged to drink plenty of water when using marjoram.

Marjoram is a good seasoning to use in spaghetti sauce, tomato dishes, and on poultry. Make sure you use well chopped leaves and toss the stems out.

20. Fennel

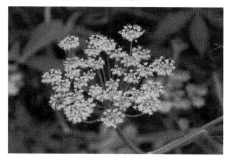

Fennel has natural diuretic properties and stimulates increased urination. It works first by helping remove uric acid from the body tissues and can help flush excess uric acid through the kidneys. By removing toxins, it can help decrease the inflammation in the body caused by gout.

Fennel has a sweet and licorice-like flavor, but it goes well in both sweet and savory dishes. You can use the entire plant, from the bulb to the leaves. Saute the bulb with onions and vegetables, sprinkle the leaves into a salad, or use leaves in sweet baked goods.

A Word of Caution with Spices for Gout

- Be sparing when you use a spice for the first time. Add a small amount and allow to simmer. Taste test after a few minutes then add a little more at a time. You really only need to start with a half-a-teaspoon, and work up to a full-teaspoon, if you desire. This is especially important if you are using a red pepper or cayenne based pepper. Cayenne really only needs to be added in "dashes."

- When using spices, try to find whatever you can fresh. Check the produce aisle to see if they have the spice available. If not, then look for a fresh chopped "jar version." As a last resort, it is okay to use the dehydrated version. Actually, some healthy antioxidants concentrate when dried and may be more powerful than fresh.

- Spices work well to compliment foods used as; rubs, liquid marinades, sprinkled on foods, tossed with pasta, used in soups/stews, or stirred into sauces. Since spices are "food grade" health supplements you can usually use any amounts you like, unless otherwise advised by your doctor.

Spices are mostly considered "low-purine" foods and most won't convert to or increase uric acid levels. There are some spices that may actually irritate and worsen gout. If you have high uric acid levels or are in an active phase of gout, you may want to avoid:

Poppy Seeds

Poppy seeds are extremely high in purines. They have about 170 mg per ½ cup. They are commonly used in baked items like; muffins, bread, bagels, and cakes. It is strongly advised not to use or eat poppy seeds with high uric acid levels or during an acute gout flare.

Sesame Seeds

Sesame is slightly lower in purines, but still over the recommended amount. Sesame seeds have around 60 mg of purines per ½ cup. They are commonly used in Asian and Middle Eastern foods. They can be used as an anti-inflammatory for arthritis sufferers, but it may trigger a gout flare. It is recommended to stay within moderate amounts if you choose to use sesame in cooking.

Pumpkin Spice

Pumpkin spice is the lowest purine containing spice, weighing in at only 44 mg per ½ cup. Since you may only use a few teaspoons, this spice may be okay. However, it is still advised to use this spice sparingly.

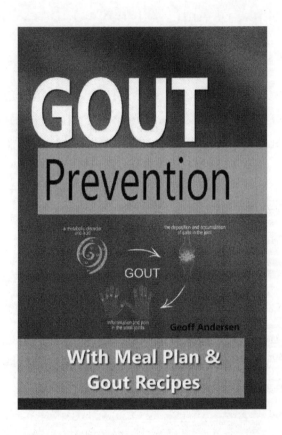

An informative book on the subject of gout, you may be interested in.

Recipes For Gout Relieving Foods Using Spices

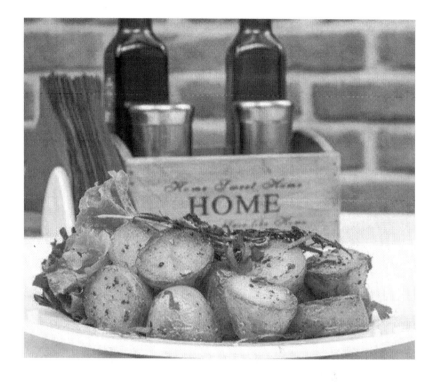

Using spices for gout relief can be easier than you think. These simple low-calorie recipes are quick to make with few ingredients for a busy lifestyle. Try these fast and easy meals to help relieve gout symptoms:

Soups and Starters

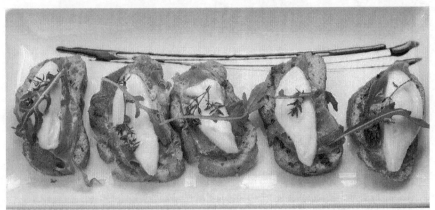

Kicking off a meal with a starter can awaken those taste buds and get them ready to taste the deliciousness of the main course. Starters can also calm hunger pains, while we wait for our meal to be ready. Some starters and soups are enough for a light meal or main course. Here are some helpful recipes to begin your mealtime, using spices that help alleviate gout symptoms.

Curried pumpkin carrot soup

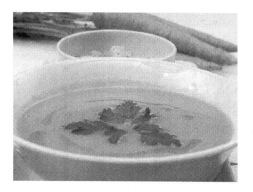

Soups can make a hearty meal that heals and warms your sore and aching joints. The flavor of this quick meal is both savory with a touch of sweetness. It pairs well with a chunk of crusty bread and good leftover the next day.

Ingredients

3 c.	**Pumpkin, Peeled and Cubed**
1 ½ c.	**Carrots, Peeled and Sliced**
1	**Potato, Peeled and cubed**
½	**Onion, Chopped**
½ c.	**Shallots, Chopped**
1 Tbsp.	**Ginger, Grated**
2 Tsp.	**Curry Powder**

2 Tsp.	Canola Oil
3 c.	Chicken Broth, Low-Sodium
½ Tsp.	Salt
¼ c.	Heavy Cream, if desired

Instructions

Heat Oil in large Skillet. Saute onion and shallots until tender and cooked. Pour in chicken broth and add potato, carrots, curry, and ginger. Simmer for 5 to 10 minutes. Add pumpkin and salt to taste. Cook 30 minutes until vegetables are soft. Use a whir blender to puree. You can add a dash of heavy cream at the very end of cooking if you like.

Stinging Nettle Pesto

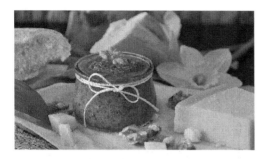

Pesto is a tart, nutty sauce that can be eaten on crusty bread, over pasta, or even as a marinade for chicken or fish. All the ingredients go straight into the blender and pulsed to the consistency you like. You can store any sauce in the fridge for up to a week and heat it up as needed.

Ingredients

6 c.	**Stinging Nettle, Raw and Packed**
½ c.	**Pine Nuts, Toasted**
2	**Garlic Cloves, Peeled**
1 c.	**Parmesan Cheese, Small Chunks or Grated**
3 Tbsp.	**Lemon Juice**
½ c.	**Extra Virgin Olive Oil**

Instructions

Throw Nettle, nuts, garlic, and cheese into blender and pulse until chopped well. Add in Lemon juice and olive oil in small batches and pulse. Continue to pulse until it reaches the consistency you like. Empty into pan and heat to use over pasta or place in a serving bowl to be used as a dip for bread or crackers. You can even use some over the top of steamed veggies.

Spring Mix Greens with Fennel Bulb

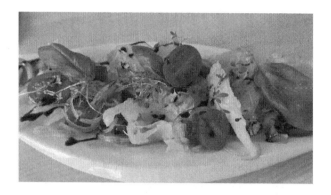

This light salad combines the sweet and crisp touches of spring mix greens and the "anise-like" flavor of fennel bulb. It works well as a first course or even with grilled chicken on top as a dinner salad. It only takes minute to toss up and works well with a vinegarette.

6 c.	**Spring Mix Greens**
3 Bulbs	**Fennel, chopped**
½ c.	**Cranberries, Dried**
1 Tbsp.	**Garlic, Minced**
3 Heads	**Radicchio, Chopped and Cored**
½	**Purple Onion, Thinly Sliced**
1 c.	**Pecans or Walnuts**

1 ¼ Tsp.	Sea Salt
¼ c.	Apple Cider Vinegar or Balsamic
¼ c.	Red Wine Vinegar
1 c.	Extra Virgin Olive Oil

Instructions

In a large bowl, mix together spring mix, radicchio, and fennel. Toss in cranberries and nuts. In medium size bowl, mix together olive oil, vinegar, salt, and garlic. Toss dressing with salad and top with a few berry tomatoes.

Pickled Cucumber Salad

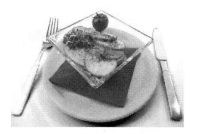

Cucumber salad can be a refreshing starter with your lunch or dinner. Most people will remember this on their grandmother preparing this light salad in the fridge. It really is as easy as she made it look and can be just as tasty.

Ingredients

3	Cucumbers, Peeled and Sliced Thin
¼ c.	Sweet Onion, Chopped
1 Tsp.	Sea Salt
¼ c.	Sugar
⅛ c.	Water
¼ c.	White Vinegar or Apple Cider Vinegar
½ Tsp.	Celery Seed

Instructions

Lay cucumbers out on paper towel and sprinkle with salt. Allow to rest for 40 minutes to 1 hour. Lay another paper towel over cucumbers and press down to squeeze out excess water. Place in large bowel. Sprinkle with celery seed and toss in onion.

In a separate bowl, stir together water, sugar, and vinegar. Pour over cucumber mixture and stir. Place in refrigerator to marinate for 1 hour.

Pico de Gallo Salsa

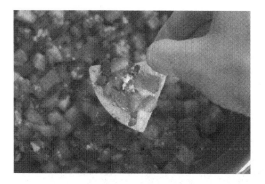

The key to the best salsa is, cilantro. Chopped into aromatic tasty bits and tossed with tomatoes, this can be a refreshing addition to any meal or great as a snack. It is good chopped up fresh or even the next day. You can use it on tacos, chips, as a marinade, or over some spicy enchiladas.

Ingredients

10-12	Roma Tomatoes, Diced
1	Sweet Onion, Chopped
2 Seeded	Jalapeno Peppers, Cored and
1 Bunch	Cilantro
1	Lemon, Juiced
2 Cloves	Garlic, Crushed
1 Tsp.	Sea Salt
½ Tsp.	Black Pepper

Instructions

Dice Tomatoes and add to large bowl. Mix in chopped onion, chopped jalapeno, and cilantro. Sprinkle in salt, pepper, and garlic. Juice lemon into bowl and stir. Allow to sit for 20 to 30 minutes and then enjoy!

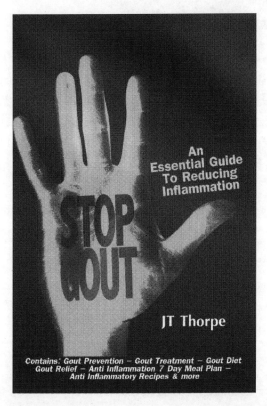

Another book on Gout you may be interested in.

Main Dishes

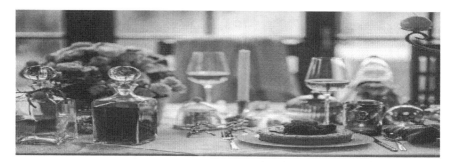

The main dish is the proverbial "star of the show," giving you the largest portion of the meal. These dishes were designed to be tasty, healthy, and satisfying. The use of spices make for some exciting flavor combinations when paired with sauteed fruits, vegetables, or sitting atop a bed of greens.

Pork Chops with Chopped Basil and Peaches

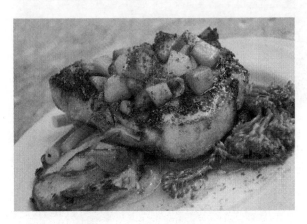

Wondering what to do with those pork chops? There are many exciting and tasty recipes for pork. Surprisingly, they work well with a number of spices! This recipe combines peaches, with fresh chopped basil to tantalize your taste buds and help with gout symptoms.

Ingredients

2- 4	**Pork Chops**
2 Tbsp.	**Extra Virgin Olive Oil**
3	**Peaches, Cut and Pitted**
2 Tsp.	**Lemon Zest**
2 Tbsp.	**Lemon Juice**
1 Tsp.	**Sugar**
½ Tsp.	**Sea Salt**

Pinch	**Red Chili Flakes**
2 c.	**Spinach**
1 Tbsp.	**Butter**
¼ c.	**Basil, Fresh and Chopped Rough**
¼ Tsp.	**Black Pepper, Ground**

Instructions

Sprinkle pork chops with salt and pepper. Heat olive oil in skillet and brown pork chops. Allow to sear 4 minutes on each side. Make sure internal temp reaches 145 degrees with meat thermometer. Take out of pan and set aside. Cover with foil.

Add lemon zest, peaches, sugar, chili flakes and salt to drippings in skillet. Saute lightly about 3 to 5 minutes. Line plates with spinach and place pork chops over. Any juice that ran off pork chops onto holding plate, pour into skillet over the peaches. Add lemon juice and butter to skillet with peaches. Saute for another 3 to 5 minutes. Add basil and allow to reduce. Top pork chops with sauce from pan.

Coriander Chicken

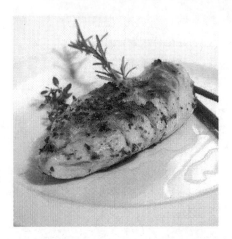

This tangy, spicy chicken recipe combines coriander with turmeric, and ginger. Three key spices that help with gout. It can be served up with couscous, risotto, or even steamed red potatoes on the side. The chicken can be cooked right away or place in the sauce to marinate overnight.

Ingredients

2 lbs.	Chicken Thighs or Breasts, Cubed
5-6 Cloves	Garlic, Crushed
1 Tbsp.	Ginger, Peeled/Chopped
4 Tbsp.	Water
1 Tsp.	Coriander Seeds, Ground
1	Green Pepper, Seeded and Chopped

½ Tsp.	Cayenne Pepper
2 Tsp.	Cumin, Ground
½ Tsp.	Turmeric Powdered
1 Tsp.	Sea Salt
¼ c.	Lemon Juice
3 Tbsp.	Olive Oil

Instructions

Heat olive oil in skillet and brown chicken. Take out of pan and set aside. Place garlic into pan and saute. Add ginger and saute. Add in Turmeric, coriander, green chili, cayenne, cumin, and salt. Saute for 1 to 2 minutes. Place chicken into pan with water and lemon juice and simmer for 15 minutes.

Sauce as marinade: In medium bowl, stir together olive oil, water, and lemon juice. Add garlic, ginger, salt, and spices. Place chicken in zip bag and pour marinade over. Place in fridge overnight. The next day, heat 3 Tbsp. Olive oil in pan and brown chicken. Remove chicken and set aside. Pour marinade out of bag and heat to boiling. Add chicken bag to pan and simmer until sauce is reduced. (Make sure sauce boils before eating to prevent food illness).

Glazed Ham with Clove

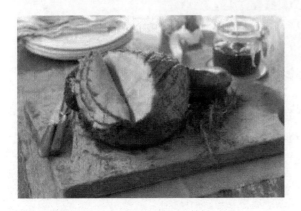

A glazed ham with clove can be a tender and succulent meal. A big enough piece of ham can give you leftovers for sandwiches, all while giving you the benefits of clove for gout relief. In this recipe, you will grind the clove powder and use it in the glaze. Making diagonal slices in the meat will allow the clove oil to both flavor the ham and infuse into the meat.

Ingredients

10 to 12 lb.	Ham, Boneless
¼ c.	Honey
1/2 c.	Brown Sugar
2 Tbsp.	Cloves, Ground
1 Tbsp.	Apple Cider Vinegar

Instructions

Preheat oven to 350 degrees.Take ham and make diagonal cuts about ¼ inch deep into meat, crisscrossing to form diamonds. Mix together; honey, brown sugar, clove powder, and vinegar in bowl. Use glazing brush to cover ham with glaze. If glaze is too thick, thin with orange juice 1 Tbsp. at a time.

Place in pan and cover with foil. Allow to roast for 1 hour. Open oven and carefully remove foil. Brush ham with glaze to coat again and cover with foil. Roast for 30 minutes and then spoon remaining glaze over the top. Leave foil off and turn oven up to 400 degrees and roast for a final 10 to 15 minutes until glaze is browned.

Chicken Tacos with Pico de Gallo

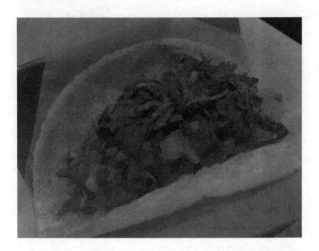

When you're craving mexican, chicken tacos spiced up with a little cayenne in the taco seasoning and topped with fresh pico de gallo is sure to satisfy. The chicken can be cooked up quickly that day, and salsa made the day before. Both the cayenne and the cilantro will help relieve gout symptoms and give your food that unique mexican flavor.

Ingredients

1 lb.	Chicken Breasts, Boneless, Skinless
2 Tbsp.	Garlic Powder
2 Tbsp.	Paprika
1 Tbsp.	Sea Salt
2 Tsp.	Cayenne Pepper

1 Tbsp.	Thyme
1 Tbsp.	Black Pepper, Ground
1 Tbsp.	Cumin
1 Tbsp.	Lime Juice
2 Tbsp.	Extra Virgin Olive Oil

Instructions

Slice chicken breasts into thin strips. Mix together spices with lemon juice and add chicken to bowl and coat. Heat olive oil in skillet and brown chicken strips until done. Pour seasoning into pan and stir. Allow chicken to simmer for 5 to 10 minutes, stirring during cooking to prevent sticking. Serve in Flour taco size tortillas topped with pico de gallo salsa (recipe above).

Sides

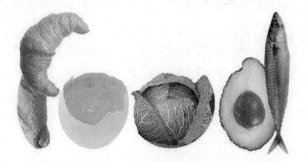

Side-dishes help balance your meal and compliment the protein that you're serving. It's important to choose foods from a variety of food groups and try to use foods from a variety of colors for the best nutrition. Careful spice choices can really bring out the flavors of your vegetables and add even more color to make your plates appealing.

Sweet Carrots with Fresh Marjoram

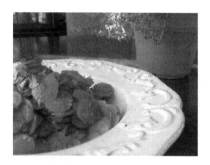

Carrots are always a sweet and fresh side dish filled with healthy nutrients. Dressed up with lemon juice, fresh marjoram, and garlic gives you a flavorful addition to any meal that is both healing and tasty.

Ingredients

2 lbs.   Carrots, Cut in Slices

1 Clove   Garlic, Peeled and Minced

3 Tbsp.   Extra Virgin Olive Oil

⅓ Tsp.   Sea Salt

¼ Tsp.   Black Pepper, Ground

1 Tsp.   Natural Sugar, Granulated

2 Tbsp.   Marjoram, Fresh and Chopped (Can substitute 1 Tbsp. Dried)

4 Tsp.   Lemon Juice

Instructions

Heat olive oil in skillet and saute carrots, sugar, and garlic. Lightly salt and pepper. Saute until carrots begin to soften. Sprinkle in marjoram and simmer gently with lid on pan for 5 to 6 minutes.

Remove cover from pan and turn heat up. Saute carrots until they begin to slightly brown. Remove from heat, sprinkle with lemon juice and serve immediately.

Roasted Red Potatoes with Rosemary

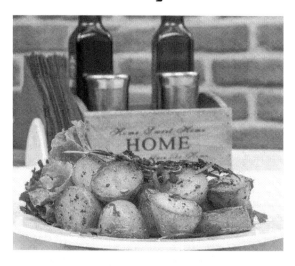

Red potatoes are a perfect pairing for meals spanning your entire day. You can toss these up with your eggs at breakfast, or enjoy them as a side for lunch or dinner. The rosemary gives you multiple benefits and a savory herb flavor for your potatoes.

Ingredients

10 to 12	Red Potatoes, Peeled or Unpeeled and halved
2 Tbsp.	Rosemary, Fresh/Minced
2 Tbsp.	Garlic, Fresh/Minced
¼ c.	Extra Virgin Olive Oil
1 Tsp.	Sea Salt

¼ Tsp.	Black Pepper, Ground

Directions

Set oven temp to 400°F and preheat for 10 to 15 mins. Place halved potatoes in large bowl and toss with; salt, pepper, rosemary, garlic and olive oil. Turn potatoes out onto a baking sheet, making sure they are well separated. Bake in oven for 30 minutes, then turn with spatula. Allow to cook 30 minutes longer until crispy and brown. Serve immediately.

Spiced Rice

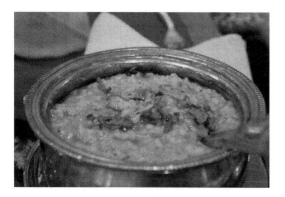

This tasty creation is infused with several of the spices known to help reduce gout symptoms and increase your body's ability to heal. This side-dish works well with a steamy bowl of lentils, tandoori chicken, or even your favorite tofu dish.

Ingredients

1 Pkg.	Basmati Rice, 10-12 Ounces
1	Onion, Small/Chopped
1 Clove	Garlic, Peeled/Chopped
1 Stick	Butter
1 Can	Vegetable Broth
½ Tsp.	Coriander Seeds
1 Stick	Cinnamon
1 Tsp.	Cumin Seeds
4-5 Pods	Cardamom
1 Tsp.	Turmeric

½ Tsp.	**Mustard Seeds, Black**
2	**Bay Leaves**
½ Tsp.	**Sea Salt**
¼ Tsp.	**Black Pepper, Ground**

Instructions

Grind coriander seeds to powder. Grind cardamom until just crushed. Crush cinnamon sticks. Grind cumin seeds. This all needs to be done separately, then mix together. You can use a mortar and pestle or electric grinder.

Take ½ stick of butter and melt in a pan. Saute the garlic and onion, then add turmeric and mustard seed to pan. Saute for 2 minutes, then add all spices from grinder mixture. Stir for another 2 minutes.

Add rice to pan and coat. Pour in broth, add salt and pepper and bring to a boil. Reduce heat and cover, allowing to simmer 15 to 20 minutes until broth is absorbed into rice. When finished, remove from heat.

Cut ½ stick of butter into cubes and add to rice. Allow it to melt into rice then fluff with a fork. Do not overstir to avoid breaking down rice. Cover with lid and allow to steep another 5 minutes with heat off. Top with bay leaves. Remind those eating to pull out any uncrushed cinnamon.

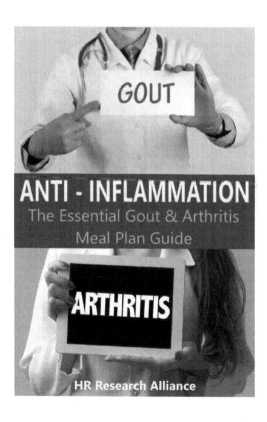

Another book on Gout You May Be interested in.

Breakfast

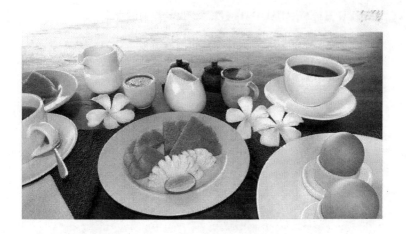

It has always been said that, "breakfast is the most important meal of the day!" Your body has just come off a 6 to 8 hour fast and needs fuel to start the day. What better way to fuel your body with energy to heal from gout, and get the benefits of spices for gout relief. Here are some quick and easy ideas to give your body a good start.

Fruited Oatmeal with Cinnamon and Flax

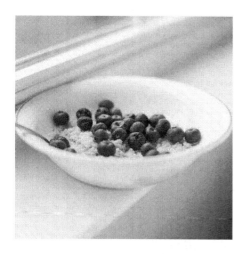

Oatmeal is a basic staple that is quick and easy for busy mornings. You can top it with basically any fruit you like. It's what is in the oatmeal that will have the most impact on your health. Add in a sprinkle of flax for antioxidants, and cinnamon for anti-inflammatory action. Plus, oatmeal is high in fiber and keeps you full until lunchtime.

Ingredients

1 c.	**Steel Cut Oats**
2 c.	**Spring Water**
¼ c.	**Milk**
½ Tsp.	**Sea Salt**

½ Tsp.	Cinnamon
1 Tbsp.	Flax Seeds, Ground to open hulls
½ c.	Fruit of your choice

Instructions

Bring water and salt to boil. Add oatmeal and milk. Allow to simmer 5 minutes if regular oats and 3 minutes if quick cook type. Turn off heat, and stir in Cinnamon and flax seeds and cover. Allow to steep another 3 to 5 minutes. Place oatmeal in bowl and top with your choice of; berries, bananas, apples, peaches, or any other fruit you like.

Spiced Wheat Pancakes

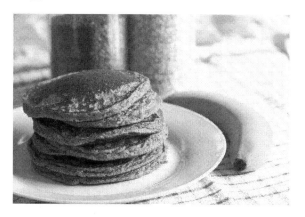

You won't even be able to tell the difference between this "healthier" version of pancakes using whole wheat flour, and the usual buttermilk pancakes with white flour. They still come out just as light and fluffy, with the added benefit of ground cloves, and cinnamon for your gout symptoms. You can even make a batch of this batter and store it in an airtight container in your fridge for up to 3 days.

Ingredients

2 c.	**Wheat Flour**
1 Tbsp.	**Baking Powder**
½ Tsp.	**Sea Salt**
½ Tsp.	**Ground Clove**
1 Tsp.	**Cinnamon**

¼ Tsp.	Nutmeg
3	Eggs, Large
2 c.	Buttermilk
½ Stick	Butter, Melted
1 Tbsp.	Sugar

Instructions

Sift together; flour, baking powder, salt, sugar, and spices in a large bowl and set aside. Melt butter in small bowl and set aside. In medium bowl whisk together; buttermilk, and eggs. Pour buttermilk mixture into large bowl with flour mixture and add melted butter. Stir gently just until batter is wet and leave some lumps. Do not overmix. Drop onto heated greased griddle and allow bubbles to form in batter before turning. Cook about 3 minutes on each side and serve right away with warm maple syrup or top with fruit.

Eggs Ranchero with Rosemary Toast

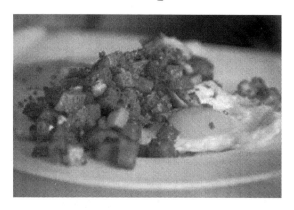

Eggs ranchero is essentially just fried eggs with a heap of salsa on top. This gives you the benefit of fresh vegetables, cilantro, and the healthy protein from eggs. Adding a piece of rosemary sourdough bread gives you something to mop up that yolk, and the healing benefits of rosemary.

Ingredients

2	**Eggs, Large**
¼ c.	**Pico de Gallo Salsa (Recipe Above)**
¼ Tsp.	**Sea Salt**
¼ Tsp.	**Black Pepper, Ground**
1 Tbsp.	**Extra Virgin Olive OIl**
2 Slices	**Sourdough Bread**

½ Tsp.	Rosemary, Crushed
2 Pats	**Butter**

Instructions

Heat oven to 325 degrees. Butter both sides of bread and sprinkle on Rosemary. Place on baking sheet in oven. Heat olive oil in skillet and crack in eggs. Fry to desired doneness and slide onto plate. Top with salsa. Check toast and remove from oven when brown on both sides, about 5 minutes. You may need to flip bread at about 3 minutes. Remove toast from oven, place on plate and garnish plate with fresh fruit if you like.

Peppermint Lemon Balm Tea and Muffins

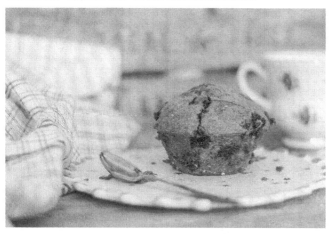

If you don't have time for a cooked breakfast, a quick alternative would be a tea containing herbs to relieve gout symptoms and a muffin. This helps fill your stomach and have some relief on board to start your day. The peppermint has properties that can help lower uric acid levels. Lemon balm is both an anti-inflammatory and has diuretic properties that helps to flush out toxins like, uric acid.

To make Tea:

Take 2 tablespoons of fresh peppermint and 2 Tablespoons dried lemon balm and add to small teapot. Pour 2 cups boiling water over and allow to steep for 5 to 10 minutes. Makes 2 cups of tea.

Enjoy with your favorite muffins either homemade or bakery fresh.

Belgian Waffles with Lavender Cream and Berries

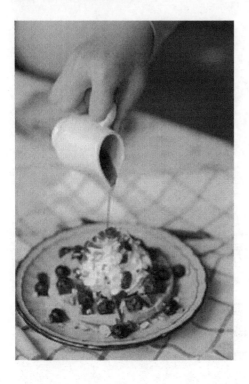

Waffles are always a hit at breakfast. They are sweet and filled with energizing carbs to refuel your body. Infusing cream with lavender can help you reduce gout symptoms and makes a beautiful presentation when topped with fresh fruit.

Waffle Ingredients

2 c.	Flour
½ Tsp.	Sea Salt, Fine
4 Tsp.	Baking Powder
¼ c.	Raw Sugar, Granulated
2 c.	Milk
½ c.	Oil
2 Large	Eggs, Separated

Instructions

Sift together; flour, baking soda, and salt. Add in sugar. In a separate bowl, whisk together egg yolks and milk. Pour in oil and stir. In another bowl, beat the egg whites until they form stiff peaks.

Pour milk mixture into flour mixture and stir. Fold egg whites into mix. Spray waffle iron with cooking spray and cook waffle batter ⅛ to ¼ cup at a time until brown. Top with lavender whipped cream (recipe below) and fresh fruit. You can also use real maple syrup with or without the cream.

Lavender Whipped Cream

This dreamy whipped topping can be used on waffles, pancakes, or even desserts. It has a slight hint of fragrant lavender and lightly sweet.

Ingredients

1 c.   **Heavy Whipping Cream**

1 c.   **Berries (blueberries, raspberries, strawberries, etc.)**

2 Tbsp.   **Sugar, Superfine**

2 Tsp.   **Lavender, Dried and Crushed with mortar and pestle**

Instructions

Add heavy cream and lavender to saucepan and simmer lightly for 2 to 3 minutes. Pour through strainer and toss lavender. Place bowl in fridge and chill until cold. Pour into a cold metal or glass bowl and whip with mixer until peaks form. Add sugar a little a a time and beat. Place back into fridge and chill before use. (Best made the night before)

Desserts

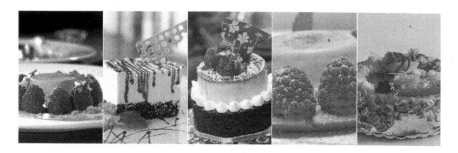

Desserts aren't always sinful, as a matter of fact, they can be quite healthy if the right ingredients are used. These tasty treats are a great way to end your meal and give your body a boost of gout fighting nutrients.

Snickerdoodles

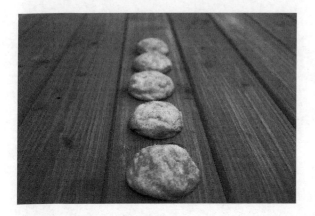

These warm cookies are always a hit and easy to make. They combine a simple sugar cookie recipe and coated with cinnamon sugar. You can make the basic dough the night before and chill for best baking results. A little patience and you get the perfect chewy inside and crispy outside. The cinnamon will help benefit gout symptoms and satisfy sweet cravings!

Ingredients

2 ½ c.	Flour
1 ½ c.	Raw Sugar, Granulated
1 Tsp.	Baking Soda
¼ Tsp.	Sea Salt, Fine
2 Tsp.	Cream of Tartar
2 Tbsp.	Sugar, Granulated (Set Aside for Topping)

1 Tbsp.	Cinnamon
1 c.	Butter
2 Large	Eggs
1 Tbsp.	Vanilla Extract

Instructions

Heat oven to 350 degrees. In large bowl, sift together; flour, cream of tartar, baking soda, and salt. In separate bowl; cream butter, sugar, vanilla, and eggs. Blend all ingredients together and turn out onto plastic wrap. Wrap tightly and place in fridge for up to 2 hours. In large zip bag, mix together sugar and cinnamon. Remove dough from fridge and form into 1 to 2 inch balls. Place in zip bag and shake to coat with cinnamon mixture. Place on cookie sheet and bake 8 to 10 minutes until lightly browned.

Peppermint White Chocolate Mousse

1 ½ c.	Heavy Cream
12 oz. Sweet	White Chocolate Chips, Semi-Sweet
½ Tsp.	Peppermint Extract
2 Tbsp.	Peppermint Candy, Crushed

Instructions

Place ¾ of the heavy cream in a saucepan and heat slowly while whisking. Do not boil. Turn off heat when hot and pour in chocolate chips. Stir well until all chips are melted. Add peppermint extract and stir.

Cool in fridge until completely cooled. In a separate bowl, beat remainder of heavy cream until stiff peaks form. Take cooled chocolate mixture from fridge and stir into beaten cream very gently. Spoon into ramekins and top with crushed candies.

Carrot Cake with Lavender Cream Cheese Frosting

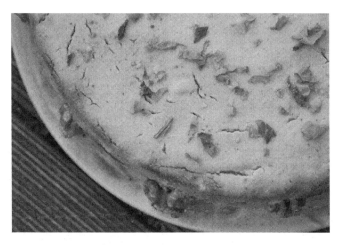

Carrot cake is always a favorite for dessert. This version incorporates both cinnamon and lavender for two gout relieving ingredients and doesn't skimp on deliciousness! Make the frosting up the night before so the lavender oils can soak in nicely. Organic ingredients will give your cake a "fresh from the garden" taste to please your tastebuds.

Cake Ingredients

2 c.   **Organic Cake Flour/or All Purpose Flour**

1 c.   **Organic Raw Sugar**

2 c.   **Carrots, Peeled/Grated/Water Squeezed Out**

2 Tsp.   **Baking Soda**

1 Tsp.	Baking Powder
½ Tsp.	Sea Salt
2 Tsp.	Cinnamon, Ground
½ Tsp.	Nutmeg, Ground
½ Tsp.	Lavender, Dried
1 Tbsp.	Orange Zest
2 Large	Eggs, Cage-Free Organic
¾ c.	Extra Virgin Olive Oil
2 Tsp.	Organic Vanilla Extract

(½ c. Chopped Walnuts if desired)

Cake Instructions

Heat oven to 350 degrees. Grease 4 cake pans (about 5") or 2 eight inch pans. Sift together; flour, baking soda, baking powder, salt, and spices. Cream together; eggs, sugar and vanilla. Stir in vanilla and oil and mix into flour mixture. Make sure carrots are well-drained by pushing into strainer and squeezing in towels. Stir in carrots and lavender.

Pour batter into pans and bake 20 to 30 minutes until toothpick comes out clean in center. Cool on racks and frost with frosting below.

Frosting Ingredients

3 Tbsp.	Butter, Organic/Unsalted
3 oz.	Cream Cheese
2 c.	Powdered Sugar, Organic
2 Tsp.	Vanilla Extract, Organic
2 Tbsp.	Lavender, Dried/Crushed

Instructions

Soften butter and cream cheese to room temperature while mixing and baking cake. Place into mixing bowl and blend with vanilla until smooth. Mix in powdered sugar a few tablespoons at a time. Sprinkle in lavender and mix well. Spread on cakes when cool. You can save a few sprigs of fresh lavender with purple flowers to garnish the cake if you like.

Beverages

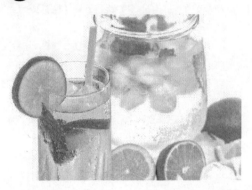

A warm cup of tea on a rainy day or a cool drink on a hot day can refresh you and help with your gout symptoms. You can take a number of beverages and add spices that help relieve gout symptoms. The possibilities are endless, but here are a few to help you get started.

Cinnamon Licorice Tea

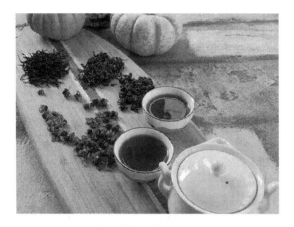

Make sure you ask your doctor before consuming licorice, especially if you have high blood pressure

Cinnamon licorice tea can be taken either hot or cold and has two great spices for gout relief. Brew this up and keep it in your fridge to take up to 2 cups a day.

Ingredients

1 Tbsp.　**Green or Black Tea**

1 Tbsp.　**Licorice, Ground**

1 Tsp.　**Cinnamon, Crushed**

Instructions

Take tea, licorice and cinnamon and mix together. Place in tea bag or strainer and pour one cup of boiling water over. Steep for 5 minutes and remove tea. Stir in honey to taste, if you like. Drink one to two cups daily.

Peppermint Iced Tea

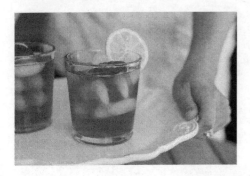

Peppermint iced tea is a refreshing drink for any kind of day whether hot or even rainy. The peppermint can relieve your gout symptoms and give your body a cool sensation that soothes pain. You can even take some of the brewed tea and use it as a compress on sore joints.

Ingredients

6 Tbsp.	**Peppermint Leaves, Fresh or Dried**
2 Sprigs	**Peppermint, Fresh**
6 c.	**Boiling Water**
3 c.	**Ice**

Instructions

Place tea in saucepan and add 6 cups boiling water. Cover pan and allow to steep for 10 to 15 minutes. Remove lid and cool down with peppermint in pan. Strain into 2 quart pitcher over ice cubes. Top with sprigs of peppermint. Serve in iced glasses.

Clove Tea

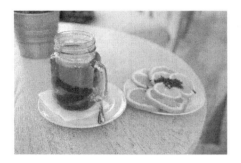

Cloves are a strong and spicy herb that actually make delicious herbal tea. You won't have to use as much as other herbs or steep it as long to get the flavor. It works well hot or cold and gives relief to gout pain, while quenching your thirst.

Ingredients

1 Tsp.   **Clove, Ground**

1 c.   **Boiling Water**

2-3 Slices Orange

Instructions

Stick to about 1 teaspoon of clove or the tea may come out too potent. You can adjust the amount to your taste after you try it a few times. Take the clove and place in tea bag or strainer. Pour boiling water over tea and steep for about 5 minutes or to your taste. Remove tea and garnish with orange slices.

Gout 10 day Meal Plan

Working in spices to your weekly meal plan can help you get the most from the foods you eat while you are healing from gout. It can also help you maintain your ability to fight off and prevent future gout attacks.

All you really need to do is take note of the above spices that can help you. Add a sprinkle of cinnamon to your toast or oatmeal everyday, or drop some lemon balm into your smoothie. You can also end your meal with a cup of hot clove tea.

The recipes above will get you started, but try to find new recipes to give yourself some variety. This way, you are eating healthy meals that help combat inflammation, pain, and elevated uric acid level.

Breakfast – Lunch – Dinner

Day 1
Oatmeal with Cinnamon
Fresh Blueberries
Toast
Curried pumpkin carrot soup
Chicken Salad Sandwich Glazed Ham with Clove
Sweet Carrots with Fresh Marjoram
Carrot Cake with Lavender Cream Cheese Frosting

Day 2
Eggs Ranchero with Pico de Gallo
Toast
Ham Sandwich
Pickled Cucumber Salad
Grilled Steak
Pickled Cucumber Salad

Day 3
Spiced Wheat Pancakes
Sausage Spring Mix Greens with Fennel Bulb
*Grilled Chicken Breast Pork Chops with Chopped Basil
and Peaches*
Rice or Potato

Day 4
Scrambled Eggs
Peppermint Lemon Balm Tea and a muffin Pork Chops
with Chopped Basil and Peaches   Stinging Nettle
Pesto over Pasta
Baguette

Day 5
Cold Cereal
Toast
Clove Tea   Stinging Nettle Pesto over Pasta
Green Salad Chicken Tacos with Pico de Gallo

Day 6
Belgian Waffles with Lavender Cream and Berries
Ham Slice   Chicken Tacos with Pico de Gallo
Grilled Salmon
Roasted Red Potatoes with Rosemary

Day 7
Fruited Oatmeal with Cinnamon and Flax
Fried egg (optional)
Toast
Spring Mix Greens with Fennel Bulb topped with Grilled
Salmon
Curried pumpkin carrot soup
Baguette
Snickerdoodles

Day 8
Scrambled Eggs with Pico de Gallo
Fresh Strawberries
Toast
Fresh Fruit
Spring Mix Greens with Fennel Bulb
Grilled Chicken Breast
Coriander Chicken
Spiced Rice
Peppermint White Chocolate Mousse

Day 9
Cinnamon Licorice Tea
Muffin of Choice
Coriander Chicken
Green Salad
Fresh Fruit
Pork Chops with Chopped Basil and Peaches
Sweet Carrots with Fresh Marjoram

Day 10
Egg Sandwich on Rosemary Toast
Peppermint Tea   Curried pumpkin carrot soup
Baguette
Pizza Night!
Peppermint White Chocolate Mousse

This meal plan is designed to make some things in larger batches and use some meals for leftover lunches. This helps you save time and get the most out of your meals. Make up large batches of salsa for marinades, toppings and snacking with chips. Mousse, cookies and cakes will all keep for up to two weeks if wrapped and stored properly.

You can also mix and match this menu with your own personal weekly menu to give you more meal options. You can even experiment with the spices above in your own favorite dishes.

Try to include a variety of beverages to help balance your diet. Good ideas include:

- Flax Milk
- Juices (cranberry, orange, grapefruit, and apple)
- Spring Water
- Herbal Tea
- Mineral Water
- Almond or Rice Milks
- Coconut Water

Try to avoid caffeinated beverages like coffee and caramel colored soda, they can increase the risk of kidney stones. To help flush uric acid, increase your fluid intake. Water is always best and you should try to get at least 2 liters a day.

Lifestyle Changes For Preventing Gout

Along with a healthy diet incorporating the spices listed above, there are several lifestyle changes you can do to help you recover from gout and prevent future flares. Try these practices every day, and exercise as much as you can tolerate without too much pain. Here are some good lifestyle changes for living with gout:

Increase Fluid Intake. It is recommended that you try to drink at least 2 liters of water daily, more or less depending on your doctor's recommendations. A good way to measure out water intake, is to clean out a 2 liter soda bottle and fill it for the day. If you drink it all you can always refill it. Try to use filtered or spring water if you can. Keep a portable water bottle with you at all times during the day and sip often. If you take water in the car, try to use a glass or metal water bottle.

Balance Your Diet. In addition to the recipes and meal plan above, try to include plenty of; fresh vegetables, fresh fruits, whole grains, lean proteins, healthy fats, and a few servings of calcium foods daily. Reduce your intake of starchy carbohydrates, sugar, and high fructose corn syrup. Try switching to raw unrefined sugar and/or honey.

Reduce or Avoid Alcohol. Alcohol can increase gout symptoms, elevate uric acid levels, and increase the risk of kidney stones. Beer is especially high in purines that can raise your uric acid levels. New studies show that beer should be avoided, but less than two glasses of wine daily may be safe. Other spirits may increase the risk of gout. If you drink more than two alcoholic beverages daily, it is important to discuss this with your doctor and get help if you need it.

Focus on Healthy Fats. Not all fats are bad. Try to get healthy fats from; avocado, extra virgin olive oil, nuts, and coconut oil. Reduce your intake of; animal fats, corn oil, margarine, trans and saturated fats, and shortening. This will help speed up weight loss and has protective benefits to your cardiovascular system, which can indirectly be affected by gout.

Try To Lose Excess Weight. Obesity and extra weight not only increases your risk of gout, but can worsen acute flares. In the meal plan above, you can always skip desserts and add more leafy greens to your diet, if needed. Being overweight with gout puts excess strain on your hips, knees, and feet, and can make walking very difficult. Eating a diet high in foods that cause weight gain may be high in purines and raise your uric acid levels. Getting on a healthy gout diet, even if you are only at risk may reduce your chances of an acute flare.

Avoid Purine Foods. Avoid foods that are high in purines. Purines convert into uric acid, this causes the uric acid crystals that irritate the joints during a gout flare. Some high purine foods include:

- Liver, Brain, Kidney, and other organ meat

- Mackerel, Anchovy, Mussels, Fish Eggs, Sardines, and Scallops (Salmon is a good seafood if eaten in moderation)

- Gravy, Cream Sauces, Cheese Sauce

- Rich Foods (foods made with meat fats)

- Cured Meats (Bacon, lunch meats, hot dogs, pork chops, cured ham)

- Lamb

- Venison, Bison, Moose Meat

- Asparagus (Mild Risk)

- Spinach (Mild Risk)

Naturally, you won't want to completely avoid some foods. If they are a mild or low-risk food, you may want to just reduce your consumption.

Increase Vitamin C Intake. While it has been shown in recent studies that vitamin C may not have any benefits in reducing uric acid levels as once thought, it may help with gout prevention. If you are at risk for gout, try to get more than 250 mg and 1500 mg of vitamin C daily from foods like; oranges, kiwi, broccoli, and other citrus fruits. One thing that citric acid may help with is reducing the build-up of crystal forming materials in the kidneys during a gout flare.

Increase Potassium Intake. Foods high in potassium may also help stop uric acid crystals from forming in the urine. Increasing potassium foods like; oranges and orange juice, bananas, potatoes, and lima beans. The type of potassium that can help reduce uric acid crystals in urine is either citrate or maleate. You can also ask your doctor about an over-the-counter supplement if he or she thinks you may need it.

Try Lemon Juice Daily. A daily squeeze of lemon in your water can be a very powerful antioxidant. This can help neutralize the uric acid that runs through the kidneys, helping it pass from the body more effectively. Lemon juice starts cleaning out the blood that runs through your liver removing toxins there and then on to the kidneys. Just use caution if you have any digestive disorders or any form of acidosis.

Use Low-Fat Dairy Products or Dairy Alternatives. The lower in fat your dairy products, the better. High fat dairy products may contain higher purine levels. Try to use low-fat or skim milk and cheese. If you can, try to switch to dairy alternatives. Just avoid soy products, they tend to raise uric acid levels. Good alternatives include; almond milk, flax milk, or coconut milk. There are also some delicious vegan cheeses made from nuts.

Exercise 3 Times A Week. During an acute flare, you may be stuck in bed for a week or even two. After the flare subsides, begin walking at a moderate pace a few times a week, as tolerated with your doctor's okay. You can also try some gentle yoga stretches when you're feeling better and light weight bearing exercises. This will help you lose any excess weight and increase the strength of your muscles around the affected joints.

If you have had a particularly severe gout flare, your doctor may recommend physical therapy to start. They can work with you to gently get your strength back and teach you exercises to use at home. You can also talk to your doctor about enrolling in a "gentle yoga" class designed for people with arthritis. While powerful advanced type yoga may overstretch the joints, gentle yoga may actually help improve stability.

Double Check Drug Interactions. Most importantly, when using any complementary or alternative medicine approaches with gout, always check for drug/herb interactions with your doctor. When you go for your doctor visits, take a list of things you are taking and eating with you so your doctor can compare them for interactions. It is also a good idea to let your pharmacy know, as well. Some spices and herbal remedies may interact with other health conditions or medications. For instance; omega-3 supplements and garlic can also have blood thinning effects and may not be appropriate if you are on blood thinning medications. Likewise, if you are on a blood thinner, some foods are high in vitamin K and may counteract the blood thinner. While certain drugs may be used for other health conditions, they may be affected by home remedies for gout. The good news is most spices that you use in cooking are considered generally safe when used in moderation.

Conclusion

Cooking with spices for gout relief can be a very healthy complement to your gout treatment plan. Meals can be planned for one person, two people, or an entire family and they are tasty enough for everyone to enjoy. Plus, you get the benefits of helping your body reduce uric acid levels, lower inflammation and feel better fast!

Always consult your doctor for your individual needs. This book is not intended to be a substitute for the medical advice of a licensed physician. The reader should consult with their doctor in any matters relating to his/her health.

We thank you, and value your comments, and reviews for this book. Please share your experience with others, so they may benefit from your knowledge on the subject. Your experiences, and thoughts, can help benefit those struggling, more than you could possibly imagine. Placing your ideas, and experiences in the review section of this book, will make it seen by others, who will benefit from your help. 5 minutes of your time, can help change someone's life for the better. Thank you.

The next section is 50 smoothie recipes for Gout Relief.

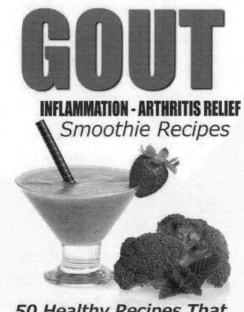

The Absolute Smoothie: Apple, Banana, Strawberry

Servings: 2

Ingredients

- 1 cup strawberries, halved
- 1 red apple, cored quartered, with skin
- ½ cup apple juice , unsweetened
- 1 banana, peeled
- 4-6 ice cubes

Directions

1. Combine ingredients in a blender. Cover and blend until smooth.

Nutritional Information (per serving)

- Calories 137
- Fat .5 g
- Carbohydrates 34.6 g
- Sugar 18.2 g
- Protein 1 g

Refreshing Classic: Oranges, Apple, Grape

Servings: 2

Ingredients

- 1 red apple, cored and quartered, with skin
- ½ cup apple juice , unsweetened
- 1 orange, peeled and separated
- 1 cup red grapes
- 4-6 ice cubes

Directions

1. Combine ingredients in a blender. Cover and blend until smooth.

Nutritional Information (per serving)

- Calories 303.9
- Fat .4 g
- Carbohydrates 77.9 g
- Sugar 51.4 g
- Protein 2.4 g

Banana Bahama Mama: Banana, Pineapple, Orange

Servings: 2
Ingredients
- 1 cup frozen pineapple chunks, unsweetened
- 1 orange, peeled and separated
- 1 banana, peeled
- ½ cup low-fat vanilla yogurt
- ½ cup coconut water
- 3-5 ice cubes

Directions
1. Combine ingredients in a blender. Cover and blend on high until smooth.

Nutritional Information (per serving)
- Calories 448
- Fat 0 g
- Carbohydrates 51 g
- Sugar 36 g
- Protein 6 g

Orange Power: Orange, Carrot, Turmeric

Servings: 2

Ingredients

- 1 orange, peeled and separated
- 1 ½ cup shredded carrots
- ½ tsp. ground turmeric
- ½ cup water*
- 4-6 ice cubes

Substitute with ½ cup apple juice, if desired.

Directions

1. Combine ingredients in a blender. Cover and blend until smooth.

Nutritional Information (per serving)

- Calories 142
- Fat 0 g
- Carbohydrates 35 g
- Sugar 22 g
- Protein 4 g

What a Plummy Pear: Plum, Pear, Blueberry

Servings: 2
Ingredients
- 1 pear, cored and chopped, with skin
- 2 plums, halved and pitted
- 1 cup frozen blueberries, unsweetened
- ½ cup low-fat blueberry yogurt
- ½ tsp. cinnamon

Directions
1. Combine ingredients in a blender. Cover and blend until smooth.

Nutritional Information (per serving)
- Calories 176.3
- Fat 1.6 g
- Carbohydrates 41.5 g
- Sugar 30.9 g
- Protein 2.6 g

Merry Berries and Plum: Cherry, Strawberry, Plum

Servings: 2

Ingredients

- 1 cup strawberries, halved
- 2 plums, pitted and halved
- 1 cup cherries, pitted
- 1 cup original almond milk, unsweetened
- 3-6 ice cubes

Directions

1. Combine ingredients in a blender. Cover and blend until smooth.

Nutritional Information (per serving)

- Calories 237
- Fat 3.4 g
- Carbohydrates 54.9 g
- Sugar 42.6 g
- Protein 4.4 g

Apple Pie: Apple, Cinnamon, Almond

Servings: 2

Ingredients

- 2 apples, cored and quartered, with skin
- 2 tbsp. creamy almond butter
- 1 cup original almond milk, unsweetened
- ½ cup low-fat plain yogurt
- ½ tsp. cinnamon
- ¼ tsp. nutmeg
- Pinch cloves
- Pinch of ginger

Directions

1. Combine ingredients in a blender. Cover and blend until smooth.

Nutritional Information (per serving)

- Calories 224.7
- Fat 10.6 g
- Carbohydrates 25.9 g
- Sugar 17.2 g
- Protein 10.1 g

Beet the Rush Smoothie: Beet, Strawberry, Raspberry

Servings: 2

Ingredients

- 1 small beetroot, trimmed and quartered
- 1 cup frozen strawberries, unsweetened
- 1 small banana, peeled
- ½ cup red raspberries
- ¾ cup orange juice

Directions

1. Preheat oven to 400° F.
2. While oven is preheating, wash and trim leaves off of beet. Cut into quarters and place on a baking sheet. Bake for 30 minutes, or until soft.
3. Combine ingredients in a blender. Cover and blend until smooth.

Nutritional Information (per serving)

- Calories 146.2
- Fat .8 g
- Carbohydrates 35.5 g
- Sugar 14.4 g
- Protein 2.5 g

Watermelon-Basil Lemonade: Watermelon, Strawberry, Basil

Servings: 2
Ingredients
- 5 cups watermelon, cubed and seeded
- 1 cup frozen strawberries, unsweetened
- ½ cup cucumber slices
- ½ cup lemon juice
- 4 fresh basil leaves

Directions
1. Combine ingredients in a blender. Cover and blend until smooth.

Nutritional Information (per serving)
- Calories 164.2
- Fat 2 g
- Carbohydrates 39 g
- Sugar 28.4 g
- Protein 3.3 g

Creamy Cantaloupe: Cantaloupe, Pineapple, Banana

Servings: 2

Ingredients

- 1 cup cantaloupe chunks
- ½ cup frozen pineapple chunks, unsweetened
- ½ banana, peeled
- ¼ cup shredded carrots
- ½ cup coconut water

Directions

1. Combine ingredients in a blender. Cover and blend until smooth.

Nutritional Information (per serving)

- Calories 102
- Fat 0 g
- Carbohydrates 25 g
- Sugar 19 g
- Protein 2 g

Peary-Cherry: Pear, Cherry

Servings: 2
Ingredients

- 1 pear, cored and chopped, with skin
- 1 small apple, cored and quartered, with skin
- 1 cup frozen cherries, pitted
- ½ cup beet juice*
- ½ almond milk, original unsweetened
- 3-5 ice cubes

Substitute with cherry or apple juice , if desired.

Directions

1. Combine ingredients in a blender. Cover and blend until smooth.

Nutritional Information (per serving)

- Calories 135.3
- Fat .8 g
- Carbohydrates 33.1 g
- Sugar 21.4 g
- Protein 1.6 g

Peaches and Green: Peach & Avocado

Servings: 2

Ingredients

- 2 ripe peaches, pitted and quartered
- 1 ripe avocado, pitted and peeled
- 1 cup vanilla almond milk, unsweetened
- ½ small banana, peeled
- 1 tbsp. creamy cashew butter*

Substitute with almond or peanut butter, if desired.

Directions

1. Combine ingredients in a blender. Cover and blend until smooth.

Nutritional Information (per serving)

- Calories 250.2
- Fat 17.1 g
- Carbohydrates 26 g
- Sugar 12.3 g
- Protein 4.9 g

Sweet Potato Pie: Sweet potato & Banana

Servings: 2
Ingredients
- 1 medium sweet potato
- ½ banana, peeled
- 1 cup vanilla almond milk, unsweetened
- 2 tbsp. creamy cashew butter*
- ½ tsp. cinnamon
- Pinch of nutmeg
- Pinch of ginger
- Pinch of allspice
- 3-4 ice cubes

Substitute with peanut or almond butter, if desired.

Directions
1. Preheat oven to 350°F.
2. While oven is preheating, wash the potato. Pierce several times with a fork before baking it in the oven for 50 minutes, or until tender. Remove peel from potato and cool.
3. Once cooled, combine ingredients in a blender. Cover and blend until smooth.

Nutritional Information (per serving)
- Calories 179.8
- Fat 9.2 g
- Carbohydrates 21.7 g
- Sugar 6.2 g
- Protein 4.7 g

Sweet Peach Tea: Peach, Green Tea

Servings: 2
Ingredients
- 2 ripe peaches, pitted
  - 1 cup water
- 1 green tea packet*
- 2 dates, pitted
- 1 small apple, cored and quartered, with skin
  - 3-4 ice cubes

Substitute with peach tea, if desired.

Directions
1. Bring 1 cup water to boil, then let cool for approximately 2 minutes, or until 175°F. Steep one green tea packet in water for 1 minute. Remove packet and let cool.
2. Combine ingredients in a blender. Cover and blend until smooth.

Nutritional Information (per serving)
- Calories 139.7
- Fat .3 g
- Carbohydrates 36.2 g
- Sugar 29.1 g
- Protein 1.3 g

Sparkling Peach Spritzer: Peach, Grape

Servings: 2
Ingredients
- ½ cup apple juice
- 1 tbsp. lime juice
- 1 ripe peach, pitted and quartered
- 1 cup seedless green grapes
- 4-5 ice cubes

Directions
1. Combine ingredients in a blender. Cover and blend until smooth

Nutritional Information (per serving)
- Calories 107
- Fat .3 g
- Carbohydrates 27.8 g
- Sugar 16.3 g
- Protein 1 g

Cherry Citrus Smoothie: Pineapple, Cherry

Servings: 2
Ingredients
- 1 cup frozen pineapple chunks, unsweetened
- 1 cup cherries, pitted
- ½ cup orange juice
- ½ cup coconut water

Directions
1. Combine ingredients in a blender. Cover and blend until smooth.

Nutritional Information (per serving)
- Calories 157
- Fat 0 g
- Carbohydrates 37 g
- Sugar 29 g
- Protein 3 g

Sunrise Smoothie: Kiwi, Watermelon, Strawberry

Servings: 2
Ingredients
- 1 cup watermelon chunks, seedless
- 1 kiwi, peeled and sliced
- ½ cup strawberries, halved
- ½ cup original almond milk, unsweetened
- 4-5 ice cubes

Directions
1. Combine ingredients in a blender. Cover and blend until smooth.

Nutritional Information (per serving)
- Calories 64.8
- Fat 1 g
- Carbohydrates 14.6 g
- Sugar 6.7 g
- Protein 1.3 g

Better Birthday Cake: Vanilla, Spinach, Banana

Servings: 2
Ingredients
- ½ banana, peeled
- 1 banana, frozen
- 2 tbsp. creamy cashew butter*
- 1 cup vanilla almond milk, unsweetened
- ½ tsp. pure vanilla extract
- 2 cups spinach

Substitute with almond butter, if desired.

Directions
1. Combine ingredients in a blender. Cover and blend until smooth.

Nutritional Information (per serving)
- Calories 214.6
- Fat 9.4 g
- Carbohydrates 30.5 g
- Sugar 16.5 g
- Protein 5.1 g

Blue Raspberry Tea: Blueberry, Raspberry, White Tea

Servings: 2
Ingredients
- 1 cup low-fat blueberry yogurt
- 1 tsp. lemon juice
- 1 cup red raspberries
- 1 cup blueberries
- 1 cup water
- 1 white tea bag
- 3-4 ice cubes

Directions

1. Bring 1 cup water to boil, then let cool for approximately 2 minutes, or until 175°F. Steep one white tea packet in water for 1 minute. Remove packet and let cool.
2. Combine ingredients in a blender. Cover and blend until smooth

Nutritional Information (per serving)
- Calories 120.7
- Fat .3 g
- Carbohydrates 27.4 g
- Sugar 14.4 g
- Protein 4.2 g

Blackberry Mango Tango: Blackberry, Mango, Honeydew

Servings: 2

Ingredients

- 1 cups frozen mango chunks
- 1 cup blackberries
- 1 cup honeydew melon chunks
- 1 cup coconut water
- 1 tsp. pure vanilla extract

Directions

1. Combine ingredients in a blender. Cover and blend until smooth.

Nutritional Information (per serving)

- Calories 108
- Fat 1 g
- Carbohydrates 25 g
- Sugar 16 g
- Protein 2 g

Mango Berry Smoothie: Mango, Blueberry

Servings: 2

Ingredients

- 1 cup blueberries
- 1 cup frozen mango chunks
- 1 cup original almond milk, unsweetened
- 1 tsp lemon juice
- 1 tbsp. raw coconut butter*
- 4-6 ice cubes

Substitute with almond butter, if desired.

Directions

1. Combine ingredients in a blender. Cover and blend until smooth.

Nutritional Information (per serving)

- Calories 155
- Fat 7 g
- Carbohydrates 24 g
- Sugar 17 g
- Protein 2 g

You've Broc-To Be Kidding: Broccoli, Blueberry, Orange

Servings: 2
Ingredients
- ¾ cup broccoli florets, de-stemmed
- 2 cups water
- 1 cup blueberries
- 1 orange, peeled and separated
- 1 cup orange juice
- 3-4 ice cubes

Directions
1. In a medium sauce pan, bring water to a boil. Boil broccoli for 7 minutes, or until tender. Remove from heat, drain, and let cool.
2. Combine ingredients in a blender. Cover and blend until smooth.

Nutritional Information (per serving)
- Calories 146.7
- Fat .6 g
- Carbohydrates 34.6 g
- Sugar 25.5 g
- Protein 3.5 g

Blackberry Cobbler: Blackberry, Almond

Servings: 2
Ingredients
- 1 ½ cups blackberries
- ½ cup original almond milk, unsweetened
- 2 tbsp. creamy almond butter
- ½ cup low-fat vanilla yogurt
- 1 tsp. cinnamon
- 1 tsp. vanilla extract
- 4-6 ice cubes
- Optional: add 1 Tbsp. raw honey for a sweeter smoothie

Directions
1. Combine ingredients in a blender. Cover and blend until smooth.

Nutritional Information (per serving)
- Calories 166.9
- Fat 9.1 g
- Carbohydrates 20.1 g
- Sugar 10.1 g
- Protein 4.3 g

Lean, Mean, and Green: Spinach, Celery, Kiwi

Servings: 2

Ingredients

- 2 cups spinach
- 2 celery stalks, chopped
- 1 kiwi, peeled
- 1 cup apple juice
- 4-6 ice cubes

Directions

1. Combine ingredients in a blender. Cover and blend until smooth.

Nutritional Information (per serving)

- Calories 96.5
- Fat .3 g
- Carbohydrates 22. 7g
- Sugar 14.1 g
- Protein 1.5 g

P. B. & Green: Banana, Peanut butter, Spinach

Servings: 2

Ingredients

- 1 large banana, peeled
- 2 tbsp. creamy peanut butter
- 2 cups spinach
- ½ low-fat yogurt, plain
- ½ cup original almond milk, unsweetened
- 4-6 ice cubes

Directions

1. Combine ingredients in a blender. Cover and blend until smooth.

Nutritional Information (per serving)

- Calories 172.3
- Fat 9 g
- Carbohydrates 21 g
- Sugar 10.3 g
- Protein 5.6 g

Very Berry Cranberry: Raspberry, Cranberry

Servings: 2

Ingredients

- 1 cup frozen cranberries
- ½ cup raspberries
- 1 small banana, peeled
- ½ cup original almond milk, unsweetened
- 2 tbsp. orange juice
- 4-6 ice cubes

Directions

1. Combine ingredients in a blender. Cover and blend until smooth.

Nutritional Information (per serving)

- Calories 127
- Fat 1 g
- Carbohydrates 28 g
- Sugar 15 g
- Protein 2 g

Feel the Beet: Banana & Beet

Servings: 2

Ingredients

- 1 medium banana, peeled
- 1 small beetroot
- 1 cup vanilla almond milk, unsweetened
- 1 tbsp. creamy peanut butter
- 3-4 ice cubes

Directions

1. Preheat oven to 400° F.
2. While oven is preheating, wash and trim leaves off of beet. Cut into quarters and place on a baking sheet. Bake for 30 minutes, or until soft.
3. Combine ingredients in a blender. Cover and blend until smooth.

Nutritional Information (per serving)

- Calories 132.8
- Fat 5.5 g
- Carbohydrates 19.4 g
- Sugar 10.8 g
- Protein 3.5 g

Super Booster Smoothie: Cranberry, Blueberry, Kale

Servings: 2

Ingredients

- 1 cup kale, raw and chopped
- 1 cup cranberry juice , unsweetened
- 1 cup frozen blueberries, unsweetened
- ½ banana, peeled
- 2 tbsp. orange juice

Directions

1. Combine ingredients in a blender. Cover and blend until smooth.

Nutritional Information (per serving)

- Calories 158.2
- Fat 1 g
- Carbohydrates 238 g
- Sugar 29.3 g
- Protein 2.3 g

Cauli-berry Smoothie: Strawberry, Cherry, Cauliflower

Servings: 2
Ingredients
- 1 cup cauliflower florets, de-stemmed
- 1 cup strawberries, halved
- 1 cup frozen cherries, pitted and unsweetened
- 1 small banana
- ½ cup low-fat plain yogurt
- 1 cup original almond milk, unsweetened

Directions
1. Combine ingredients in a blender. Cover and blend until smooth.

Nutritional Information (per serving)
- Calories 170
- Fat 1.8 g
- Carbohydrates 36.5 g
- Sugar 22.7 g
- Protein 6 g

Pumpkin Pie Smoothie: Pumpkin, Banana, Cinnamon

Servings: 2

Ingredients

- 1 cup pumpkin chunks*
- 1 banana
- 1 cup low-fat vanilla yogurt
- 1 tbsp. peanut butter
- 1 tsp. cinnamon
- Pinch of nutmeg
- Pinch of cloves
- 3-4 ice cubes
- Optional: tbsp. pure maple syrup
- Optional: ¼ cup pumpkin seeds

Substitute with 1 cup pumpkin puree, if desired

Directions

1. Preheat oven to 375°F. Bake pumpkin chunks for 50 minutes, or until soft. Peel and let cool.
2. Combine ingredients in a blender. Cover and blend until smooth.

Nutritional Information (per serving)

- Calories 212.1
- Fat 4.3 g
- Carbohydrates 33.6 g
- Sugar 21.7 g
- Protein 11.7 g

Better Bloody Mary: Tomato, Strawberry, Basil

Servings: 2

Ingredients

- 1 cup strawberries, halved
- 2 celery stalks, chopped
- ¾ cup tomato juice , unsalted
- ¼ cup water
- 3-4 basil leaves*
- 1 tsp. lemon juice
- 1/8 tsp. ground black pepper
- Pinch of cayenne pepper
- 4-6 ice cubes
- Optional: 2 celery sticks for garnish

Substitute 2 tbsp. dried basil, if desired

Directions

1. Combine ingredients in a blender. Cover and blend until smooth.
2. Optional: pour and garnish with celery sticks.

Nutritional Information (per serving)

- Calories 45
- Fat .4 g
- Carbohydrates 10.7 g
- Sugar 7.2 g
- Protein 1.5 g

Papaya Creamsicle Smoothie: Papaya, Carrot, Banana

Servings: 2
Ingredients
- 1 cup papaya, seeded and peeled
- 1 small banana, peeled
- ½ cup shredded carrots
- 1 cup coconut water
- 2 tbsp. orange juice
- 4-6 ice cubes
- Optional: 1-2 dates for a sweeter smoothie

Directions
1. Combine papaya and water; blend. Add banana, carrots, and ice. Cover and blend until smooth.

Nutritional Information (per serving)
- Calories 147.3
- Fat .5 g
- Carbohydrates 34.5 g
- Sugar 23.7 g
- Protein 2.3 g

Avo-Cacao Smoothie: Avocado, Peanut Butter, Cacao

Servings: 2

Ingredients

- 1 avocado, pitted and skinned
- 2 ½ tbsp. raw cacao powder
- 1 banana, peeled
- ½ cup low-fat vanilla yogurt
- 3 tbsp. creamy peanut butter
- ¼ cup vanilla almond milk, unsweetened
- 3-4 ice cubes

Directions

1. Combine ingredients in a blender. Cover and blend until smooth.

Nutritional Information (per serving)

- Calories 386.5
- Fat 24.5 g
- Carbohydrates 335.9 g
- Sugar 15 g
- Protein 12.5 g

Green and Blue: Avocado, Blueberry, Spinach

Servings: 2
Ingredients

- 1 ½ cup frozen blueberries, unsweetened
- 2 cups spinach
- 1 small avocado, pitted and peeled
- 1 cup original almond milk, unsweetened
- Pinch of cinnamon
- 3-6 ice cubes

Directions

1. Combine ingredients in a blender. Cover and blend until smooth.

Nutritional Information (per serving)

- Calories 206.2
- Fat 13.4 g
- Carbohydrates 23.7 g
- Sugar 9.9 g
- Protein 4.3 g

A.K.C. Champion Smoothie: Avocado, Kiwi, Cucumber

Servings: 2

Ingredients

- ½ avocado, pitted and peeled
- ½ cup apple juice
- 1 cup spinach
- 1 kiwi, peeled
- ½ cup cucumber slices
- 4-6 ice cubes

Directions

1. Combine ingredients in a blender. Cover and blend until smooth.

Nutritional Information (per serving)

- Calories 122.5
- Fat 5.9 g
- Carbohydrates 17.9 g
- Sugar 7.1 g
- Protein 2.2 g

Watermelon Sparkler: Watermelon, Cucumber, Lemon

Servings: 2

Ingredients

- 1 cup watermelon chunks, seedless
- ½ cup cucumber slices
- ½ cup green grapes
- 1 tbsp. lemon juice
- 2-3 mint leaves
- 4-6 ice cubes

Directions

1. Combine ingredients in a blender. Cover and blend until smooth.

Nutritional Information (per serving)

- Calories 57.5
- Fat .4 g
- Carbohydrates 14.3 g
- Sugar 11.1 g
- Protein 1 g

Lemon Drop Smoothie: Lemon & Cucumber

Servings: 2
Ingredients

- 1 cup low-fat vanilla yogurt
- ½ cup coconut milk, unsweetened
- ½ cup cucumber slices
- 2 tbsp. lemon juice
- 1 date, pitted*
- 4-6 ice cubes

Substitute 1 tbsp. raw honey, if desired.

Directions

1. Combine ingredients in a blender. Cover and blend until smooth.

Nutritional Information (per serving)

- Calories 102
- Fat 2.7 g
- Carbohydrates 15.8 g
- Sugar 10 g
- Protein 5.5 g

Sweet Shirley Temple: Cherry, Orange, Ginger

Servings: 2

Ingredients

- 1 cup cherries, pitted
- 1 cup orange juice
- 1 small banana
- 1 tbsp. fresh grated ginger*
- 4-6 ice cubes
- Optional: cherries for garnish

Substitute with 1 tbsp. candied ginger, if desired.

Directions

1. Combine ingredients in a blender. Cover and blend until smooth.
2. Optional: Pour and garnish with cherries on top.

Nutritional Information (per serving)

- Calories 149.3
- Fat .8 g
- Carbohydrates 36.5 g
- Sugar 20.3 g
- Protein 2.3 g

P.B & K: Pineapple, Blueberry, Kale

Servings: 2

Ingredients

- 1 cup kale, chopped
- 1 cup blueberries
- 1 cup frozen pineapple chunks, unsweetened
- 1 cup low-fat blueberry yogurt
- 4-6 ice cubes

Directions

1. Combine ingredients in a blender. Cover and blend until smooth.

Nutritional Information (per serving)

- Calories 211
- Fat 2 g
- Carbohydrates 45 g
- Sugar 32 g
- Protein 6 g

Purple Power Punch: Red Cabbage, Cherry, Blackberry

Servings: 2

Ingredients

- 1 cup frozen cherries, pitted
- 1 cup strawberries, halved
- ½ cup blackberries
- 1 cup red cabbage, chopped
- ½ cup juice orange juice
- 1 cup low-fat blueberry yogurt

Directions

1. Combine ingredients in a blender. Cover and blend until smooth.

Nutritional Information (per serving)

- Calories 247.7
- Fat 2.7 g
- Carbohydrates 53.5 g
- Sugar 41.7 g
- Protein 5.3 g

Pina Caul-ada-flour Smoothie: Cauliflower, Pineapple, Orange

Servings: 2

Ingredients

- ½ cup cauliflower florets, de-stemmed
- 1 ½ cup frozen pineapple chunks, unsweetened
- 1 cup coconut milk, unsweetened
- Optional: 2 pineapple wedges for garnish

Directions

1. Combine all ingredients in a blender. Cover and blend until smooth.
2. Optional: pour into glasses and garnish the rims with pineapple wedges.

Nutritional Information (per serving)

- Calories 89
- Fat 3 g
- Carbohydrates 17 g
- Sugar 11 g
- Protein 1 g

Hibiscus Citrus Quencher: Hibiscus Tea, Orange, Strawberry

Servings: 2

Ingredients

- 1 cup water
- 1 hibiscus tea bag
- 1 cup frozen strawberries, unsweetened
- 1 orange, peeled and separated
- 1 tsp. cinnamon
- Pinch of black pepper
- 4-6 ice cubes

Directions

1. Heat water to a boil then remove from heat. Steep hibiscus tea bag for 3-5 minutes. Remove bag and let cool.
2. Combine ingredients in a blender. Cover and blend until smooth.

Nutritional Information (per serving)

- Calories 56.8
- Fat .1 g
- Carbohydrates 14.5 g
- Sugar 9.6 g
- Protein .9 g

Spiced Orange Smoothie: Orange, Turmeric, Cinnamon

Servings: 2

Ingredients

- 2 oranges, peeled and separated
- 1 cup cantaloupe chunks, peeled
- 1 cup original almond milk, unsweetened
- ½ tsp. turmeric powder
- ½ tsp. freshly grated ginger
- ½ tsp. cinnamon
- 4-6 ice cubes

Directions

1. Combine ingredients in a blender. Cover and blend until smooth.

Nutritional Information (per serving)

- Calories 103.6
- Fat 1.5 g
- Carbohydrates 16.4 g
- Sugar 18.7 g
- Protein 2.3 g

Pineapple Zinger: Pineapple, Ginger

Servings: 2

Ingredients

- 1 cup frozen pineapple, unsweetened
- 1 small banana, peeled
- 1 tbsp. freshly grated ginger
- ½ cup low-fat peach yogurt
- ½ cup coconut water
- Pinch of cinnamon

Directions

1. Combine ingredients in a blender. Cover and blend until smooth.

Nutritional Information (per serving)

- Calories 210
- Fat 7 g
- Carbohydrates 49 g
- Sugar 25 g
- Protein 2 g

Maximum Mango Smoothie: Mango, Cayenne, Strawberry

Servings: 2

Ingredients

- 1 cup mango chunks, peeled
- ½ cup frozen strawberries, unsweetened
- 1 banana, peeled
- ¼ tsp. cayenne pepper
- Pinch of cinnamon
- Dash of lime juice
- Optional: 1 tbsp. raw honey for additional sweetness

Directions

1. Combine ingredients in a blender. Cover and blend until smooth.

Nutritional Information (per serving)

- Calories 102.8
- Fat .4 g
- Carbohydrates 26.7 g
- Sugar 18.9 g
- Protein 1 g

Lettuce Be Cherry: Romaine Lettuce, Blueberry, Cherry

Servings: 2

Ingredients

- 1 cup romaine lettuce, chopped
- ½ cup cherries, pitted
- 1 cup blueberries
- 1 cup cherry juice
- 4-6 ice cubes

Directions

1. Combine ingredients in a blender. Cover and blend until smooth.

Nutritional Information (per serving)

- Calories 157.4
- Fat .1 g
- Carbohydrates 38.7 g
- Sugar 28.1 g
- Protein 2.3 g

The Ultimate Cress: Watercress, Apple, Avocado

Servings: 2
Ingredients
- ¼ cup watercress
- ½ small avocado, pitted and peeled
- 1 small banana, peeled
- 1 apple, cored and quartered, with skin
- 1 cup apple juice , unsweetened
- 3-6 ice cubes

Directions
1. Combine ingredients in a blender. Cover and blend until smooth.

Nutritional Information (per serving)
- Calories 185
- Fat 6 g
- Carbohydrates 34.9 g
- Sugar 10.5 g
- Protein 2 g

Dressed to Dill: Cucumber, Spinach, Dill

Servings: 2

Ingredients

- 2 cups cucumber slices
- ¼ cup lemon juice
- 5 sprigs of dill
- 1 cup spinach
- 1 cup low-fat plain yogurt
- 4-6 ice cubes

Directions

1. Combine ingredients in a blender. Cover and blend until smooth.

Nutritional Information (per serving)

- Calories 100.5
- Fat 2.2 g
- Carbohydrates 14 g
- Sugar 8.7 g
- Protein 7.7 g

Black Forest Cake: Cherry, Banana, Almond

Servings: 2

Ingredients

- ½ cup spinach
- 2 small bananas, peeled
- 2 tbsp. creamy almond butter
- 1/3 cup frozen cherries, pitted and unsweetened
- 1 cup vanilla almond milk, unsweetened
- 2 tbsp. raw cacao powder, extra for garnish
- 1 tsp. cinnamon
- 1 tsp. pure vanilla extract
- 3-5 ice cubes
- Optional: fresh cherries for garnish

Directions

1. Combine ingredients in a blender. Cover and blend until smooth.
2. Optional: pour into glasses and garnish with a light dusting of cacao powder and fresh cherries.

Nutritional Information (per serving)

- Calories 225.9
- Fat 11 g
- Carbohydrates 29.9 g
- Sugar 13.6 g
- Protein 5.5 g

Spiced Carrot Cake: Carrot, Almond, Cinnamon

Servings: 2

Ingredients

- 2 small bananas
- 1 cup shredded carrots
- 1 cup vanilla almond milk, unsweetened
- 2 tbsp. creamy almond butter
- ½ tsp cinnamon
- Pinch of powdered ginger
- Pinch of nutmeg
- Optional: 1 tbsp. raw honey for a sweeter smoothie
- 4-6 ice cubes

Directions

1. Combine ingredients in a blender. Cover and blend until smooth.

Nutritional Information (per serving)

- Calories 210.4
- Fat 10.5 g
- Carbohydrates 28.2 g
- Sugar 13.4 g
- Protein 4.4 g

This Book contains information that is intended to help the readers be better informed consumers of health care. It is presented as general advice on health care. Always consult your doctor for your individual needs. This book is not intended to be a substitute for the medical advice of a licensed physician. The reader should consult with their doctor in any matters relating to his/her health. No part of this Book may be reproduced or transmitted in any form or by any means, electronic or mechanical, including photocopying, recording or by any information storage and retrieval system, without written permission from the author.